How to Make Your Toddler Sleep

Introduction

Despite their small size, toddlers can be such a huge source of joy and laughter. But if they're deprived of much needed sleep, they can be cranky and difficult, becoming a great source of stress and anxiety. That's why if you have a toddler at home, it's important that you are able to make your toddler sleep well and on time, every time.

In this book, you will learn how to put your toddler to sleep. You'll read about general strategies – those that can be applied to all age brackets – and age-specific ones. After reading this book, you'll have a much better understanding of your toddlers and will thus be able to help them go to sleep easily at night.

So if you're ready to put your toddler to sleep, turn the page and let's begin!

Table of Contents

Chapter 1: The Sleep-Deprived Toddler

When your baby or toddler is deprived of much needed quality sleep, it's going to be a bad day and night for the child. And guess what, it's not just your child that'll be sleep-deprived – you will be too! Your child's ability to get enough good sleep is therefore beneficial not just for your toddler but for you as well!

The Signs

So how do you know when your child's sleep isn't enough? Your child may exhibit any or several of the following symptoms or effects of such:

- Clumsiness or being more prone to accidents;
- Your toddler easily falls asleep (in a just a few minutes or seconds) as soon as his head touches the pillow, which isn't normal as the average time for toddlers to fall asleep is about 20 minutes;
- He finds it hard to fall asleep;
- He finds it hard to wake up in the morning;
- He finds it very hard to focus or concentrate while playing;
- He takes excessively long naps;
- He's overly talkative, with more than the usual questions or tends to engage in conversations in a frenzied manner;
- He's unusually hyperactive;
- Impatience, heightened emotional sensitivity, or frequent and powerful tantrums;
- Stubbornness or defiant behavior; or
- Unusually strong appetite.

Underlying Reasons

- There are many reasons for your toddler's inability to get a good night's sleep. Some of them aren't serious, such as:
- He's become used to sleeping late in the evening;
- He consumes sugary foods or drinks close to bed time;
- He sleeps too much during the day, especially in the late afternoon; and
- He sleeps in an uncomfortable sleeping area, e.g., uncomfortable bed and sheets, hot room, poor ventilation, noise, etc.

But there are more serious physical or medical reasons that may make it hard for your toddler to sleep well at night. These may include:

Reflux: This is more common in infants than toddlers but may occur to the latter just the same. Because some of them may have underdeveloped and weak sphincters at the top of their stomachs, the stomach's acid may leak back into the esophagus (i.e., feeding tube), which is located at the back of the mouth. This is more likely to happen when toddlers lie down on their backs during sleep. Given it's a painful sensation, it can really deprive your toddler of much needed sleep at night.

Enlarged Adenoids: Adenoids help children stave off nasal infections by trapping them in the nose so that viruses and bacteria won't be able to reach the lungs through breathing or swallowing. For most children, adenoids shrink when they start going to school and may completely disappear by the time they grow up to become adults.

It's also common for adenoids to become enlarged or swollen. However, enlarged adenoids can also lead to swollen tonsils.

And if the adenoids swell so much or are regularly infected with viruses or bacteria, it will get in the way of your toddler's sleep. Signs of this include stuffy nose that forces your toddler to breathe through the mouth instead of the nose, snoring, frequently waking up at night, and sleep apnea (stops breathing for several seconds while sleeping, making the child sleepy during the day)

Narcolepsy: This sleeping disorder's quite rare and is usually due to a particular underlying immune system-related condition.

ADHD (Attention Deficit Hyperactivity Disorder): Toddlers diagnosed with this disorder tend to have very disrupted sleeping times at night, which leads to them becoming very tired during the day and quickly falling asleep.

Autism: One of this medical condition's symptoms is settling down to sleep. It's also associated with frequent waking up in the middle of the night.

In the remaining chapters of the book, we'll be discussing different ways you can help your toddler sleep well at night using general and age-specific strategies to maximize your chances of being able to successfully help your toddler enjoy deep and restful sleep at night. We'll also tackle how to do that too when your family's on a vacation so that your family travels will be a very enjoyable experience for both your toddler and the rest of the family.

Chapter 2: Putting Your Toddler to Sleep

In case you haven't noticed, toddlers aren't like lights or appliances whose power you can just switch on and off. Usually, they become even more "active" when they're already tired, just shortly before crashing themselves to sleep.

Your toddler needs to be able to rise to developmental challenges that can arise during his growing years, such as being able to control both bodily functions and emotions. Toddlers can manage emotional stress, like when they cry when you have to leave them with a baby sitter, much better when they are well rested. And that requires being able to sleep soundly every night.

Unfortunately, not all kids are born good sleepers, and many aren't. While it's true that external factors like their sleeping environment play a crucial role in insomnia, internal or innate factors can be just as crucial too. What may complicate this even more for your toddler is that young people such as him tend to be more comfortable sleeping in the presence of people. This means toddlers like a parent to be with them in the room as they sleep. This can be quite of a dilemma since indulging them on this will give them a good night's rest but may deprive you of the same and vice versa. That's why it's crucial – for everyone's sake – you need to be able to help your toddlers to acquire the habit of lulling themselves to sleep and staying asleep throughout the night.

So how can you help him do that?

Sleep Requirements and Waking Windows

On average, preschoolers and toddlers require 13 hours of shuteye each 24 hours, which can be split into 2: 11 hours of evening sleep and 2 hours of daytime naps. While preschoolers hardly seem to need to take naps, it can be very helpful for them to sleep better at night if they do so in the afternoon.

When we talk about waking windows, we are talking about that time period during the day during which your child can stay awake without having to take a nap. For infants, the wakefulness window is substantially shorter. And as they become older, that window continues to shorten even further. If you keep toddlers awake for longer than their ideal waking window, you risk giving them a hard time settling down and relaxing at night. It may also make it more challenging for toddlers to stay awake during the later parts of the day.

On average, going to bed between 7:00 and 8:00 in the evening is desirable. It's because, in most cases, such a schedule allows them to start the day their days between 6:30 and 7:30 in the morning when they sleep an average of 11 hours at night. This window is neither too early nor too late.

Unfortunately, many parents aren't aware that extending their children's waking windows past the norm may lead to their kids having to resist the urge or need to sleep. This may lead to a condition called "nap resistance." The obvious result in this case is sleep deprivation for their children.

So if you'd like to ensure that your toddler consistently gets enough quality sleep in the evening, resist the urge to extend his waking hours beyond the norm and make sure that he sleeps on time, respectively.

Chapter 3: Minimize Sleep Disruptors

Quite often, what deprives children of quality sleep aren't the conditions present during sleeping time but what they do shortly before it. In particular, the food and drinks children eat and drink, respectively, as well as children's activities shortly before bedtime can result in shallow and easily disrupted sleep. These include:

Food Intake: Do not feed your child food and drinks that are chock full of sugar because it'll make the child hyperactive just before bedtime, which will definitely make it hard for a child to sleep.

Extra-Curricular: Don't play with your child or do other activities with him – such as watching TV or playing video games on the tablet or on your smartphone – that are stimulating because it will make your child too stimulated to fall asleep early.

Errands: Avoid working your child's sleeping time around the errands you need to do or your other family activities. Do the opposite instead – work these activities around your child's sleep time. This will allow your toddler to get much needed quality snooze time on a regular basis.

Lighting: Use soft lights in the toddler's room at night as the child winds down to sleep because bright lights hinder the production of the sleep hormone melatonin, which will make it harder to fall asleep at night. When the child is about to sleep, turn off the lights or if he/she is uncomfortable in total darkness, keep a small lamp on that will give enough soft light to appease your child enough to be able to go to sleep. This will help keep the room just dark enough to be conducive to sleeping.

Sleeping Cues

It will be too late if you only put your child to sleep when he's already acting tired. The best time to put him to bed is when he starts exhibiting sleeping cues and not when already exhausted. What do these cues look like?

In general, they include him being cranky, unable to focus his attention on anything, yawning and eye-rubbing. Observe your child carefully to discover what his unique sleeping cues are so that you won't miss them when they happen. Failure to catch those cues and act accordingly can make it much harder for him to go to sleep as, by then, he will already be frantic, jumpy, or wired.

The Importance of Consistency

To help your child sleep well easily at night, you need to make the child feel a sense of inevitability, safety and calmness. And these can be accomplished by establishing a regular routine that may involve taking a nice warm bath, bedtime story reading, kissing, prayers or blessings and bed tucking right before turning off the lights for sleep. With bedtime routines, it's important not to overdo them. Doing so may take up excess time and make your child miss his sleeping windows of opportunity and have a hard time sleeping afterward.

What if your child becomes resistant or stubborn with the routine and chooses not to go with the flow? Just try to make the clock the bad guy, instead of you! How? One way to do this is by making your child a simple chart of the steps involved in the bedtime routine, which you can post in this child's room. Each step on the chart should feature a picture of your child doing each step and a clock's time that corresponds to the time at which each of the activities must be accomplished. As you go through the bedtime routine you want to establish every night with your child, point to the relevant photos. In time, your child will gradually want to cooperate.

An even better way to do this is by giving him an incentive. You can say something like:
"Hey, it's 7:00 already! You know what? We can have an extra story to read later, just before lights out, if you finish brushing your teeth now."

That should give your child the opportunity to see you as his ally rather than a stern drill sergeant. More than that, it allows him to develop a good sense of personal responsibility and the ability to make wise choices later on.

Wind Down Early

Don't expect an easy time putting your child to bed if you abruptly stop his activities and expect him to go cold turkey! Your child needs enough time to wind down, relax and be in the mood to hit the sack. To allow for this, give your child an hour or two of quiet and calmness in order to slowly wind down into a relaxed state of mind and body that's conducive to deep and restful sleep throughout the night.

A Comfortable Sleeping Environment

As part of their normal sleep cycles, it's normal for toddlers to wake up slightly in the middle of their sleep. They usually return to a deep state of slumber relatively quickly. As a parent, what you must concern yourself with is that they don't fully wake up during those "semi" wake up moments in the middle of the night due to a feeling or sense of discomfort. To ensure this doesn't happen, it will be worth investing in a bed or mattress that makes your child sleep comfortably through those minor sleep-waking moments.

Another factor that determines how comfortable your child's sleeping environment can be is room temperature. A room that's too hot or too cold can make it uncomfortable enough to disrupt your child's sleep. During the summer months, a breezy or air-conditioned room can help your child sleep comfortably while a warm pair of PJs and nice warm blanket can make it comfortable for him to sleep during the icy months of the year.

Another factor that influences your child's ability to sleep comfortably is lighting – or lack of it. Light makes people feel awake and makes it hard for them to sleep so it's best to use soft lights in your child's room especially during the last hour or two before sleeping, as I mentioned earlier. It will also help if you make his room as dark as is comfortably possible when he's already sleeping. Light makes it hard for your child's body to produce melatonin, which is a key sleeping hormone. So keep the lights down...or off.

The Biological Clock

If you want your toddler to sleep well, his body must learn how to anticipate or expect sleep at a specific time in the evening. For most toddlers, going to sleep between 6:30 p.m. and 8:00 p.m. is the ideal.

While it may be tempting to think that sleeping later in the evening will tire your child out and make him fall asleep more easily, it won't. When he stays up late, stress hormones such as cortisol and adrenalin start kicking in due to being over-tired, which will make him do as the Energizer bunny does… keep going and going and going and going. By then, it'll be much harder for him to sleep at night. After that, you'll have a hard time sleeping due to the stress.

And when he has a hard time falling asleep, guess what? He'll wake up more frequently throughout the night and will tend to wake up earlier in the day. When that happens, expect a cranky toddler during the day. Just continue experimenting with different sleeping times until you're able to see which time is optimal in terms of minimizing or keeping your child from being all wound up.

Another way to establish a consistent sleeping routine is turning by down the lights at least one hour prior to going to bed. Coupled with calm and slow routines, it helps program your child's body and mind to anticipate falling asleep at a certain time in the evening. A consistent, slow and calm pre-sleeping routine is a very effective way to lull your child to sleep compared to one that's abrupt, such as simply putting him in pajamas and turning off the lights within 2 minutes.

The key sleeping cue to watch out for here (remember our discussion on sleeping cues?) is him starting to becoming sleepy. Once you continue letting him stay awake past this moment, his body will switch to overdrive and stimulate him with adrenaline to the point when it will be very hard, if not downright impossible, to lull him into a deep and restful sleep soon.

Don't Deny the Naps Too Soon

Most toddlers are neither emotionally nor physiologically prepared to give up their regular naps – at least not until they turn 3 years old. Thus, you might consider taking it easy on your child if he still wants to take naps throughout the day before the age of 3. If you deny the toddler that, both of you will pay a heftier price in the evening – and the following day – when your child becomes too adrenalized and cranky to sleep early.

Midnight Snacks

Particularly during those growth spurt years, toddlers need to eat midway into the night. Some of the best choices for midnight snacks that won't disrupt their sleep are calming and predictable food and drinks such as a piece of toast, a slice of turkey and a glass of warm milk. The key is to choose food and drinks that are neither stimulating nor loaded with sugar. You can move your child much better through your pre-sleep routine if you can make the child eat a snack at a table in the child's room as you read them their bedtime stories. Just make sure he brushes his teeth afterward, just before going to sleep.

If your toddler still tends to still fall asleep with a feeding bottle in hand and mouth, you should disassociate him from it. Doing so will enable him to easily go back to sleep during those slight waking moments in the middle of the night because he won't be stimulated into waking up completely as he drinks from the bottle.

Regular Exercise, Laughter, and the Great Outdoors

It turns out the old folks are right when they say that for kids to sleep more soundly at night, they need to play outdoors as much as possible and not just sit inside the house playing computer games or watching TV all the time. This is great for your child too for as long as it's not a few hours before bedtime, as it will just make your toddler too energized in the evening to the point of having a difficult time sleeping.

It's also important that your child gets to laugh often because doing so allows him to bring down his stress hormone levels. Kids who normally have a hard time falling and staying asleep at night are those that carry a lot of emotional baggage. Laughing heartily and frequently can help your toddler unload emotional baggage (if he has any) to fall deeply asleep at night.

Develop New Habits for Sleeping

You may be doing your child a disservice if you're always rocking or nursing him to sleep. Why? You're making him get used to always being with you while asleep. This may result in him always looking for you as his security blanket in order to be able to go back to sleep during those mini waking times throughout the night. And that's part of his normal sleep cycle. When you're not there, going back to sleep will be very hard or practically impossible.

Your child's pre-sleep routine may not necessarily involve rocking or nursing the toddler to sleep but may nevertheless make it hard for him to go back to sleep on his own when he wakes up slightly in the middle of the night. Thus, it's important that you help him develop new sleeping habits that will empower him to sleep soundly on his own.

It may be hard at first so it's best to do this one step at a time. For example, instead of going cold turkey and just stopping rocking him to sleep, you can start by rocking him for shorter periods of time until you completely stop doing so. It'll be very difficult to develop new sleeping habits by simply going cold turkey on the one you want to replace. It must be done, pardon the pun, in baby steps.

Don't Rush It

Speaking of establishing new and independent sleeping habits, start by holding him while he goes off to sleep but not in a lying position because that puts you at risk of falling asleep as well! To help you to relax and make the most of this bonding moment, just meditate or listen to soft music.

Once your child is accustomed to falling asleep as you hold him, you should start making him accustomed to falling asleep by simply holding his hand or placing your hand on his head or forehead. You can also choose to substitute this by using a big stuffed toy or pillow in your place. Kids often love cuddling and curling around a nice, soft stuffed animal or a pillow, although it is important to choose a toy that is safe.

When your child is already able to fall asleep simply by being touched and not held, try sitting beside your child while he falls asleep. At first, you'll need to sit really close so that your child can touch you easily when he reaches out to you.

The last frontier is when your child's able to fall asleep without any physical contact with you. You then start to move your seat slowly further and further away from your child until you're able to exit the room. In moments that your child wakes up and tries to sit up, just say, "Lie down now please...it's sleep time, it's bed time." in a monotone voice.

You can also try and do something around the room while your child falls asleep. Just make sure what you'll be doing isn't noisy or will in any way distract your child from his sleep. Doing this will give your sleeping child a sense of security with your presence in the room and your proximity. You can then begin staying outside your child's room for longer and longer periods of time until you're able to finally help your child develop the habit of sleeping independently.

On those days that your child backslides and needs your physical touch again, don't sweat it. It won't derail the overall progress for as long as it doesn't happen frequently and consecutively. Just keep at it and the independent sleeping habit will eventually be established.

Lying Down With the Child on the Adult Bed

It's easy for most toddlers, yours included probably, when parents lie down with them on their beds. This can be especially challenging for the parents because often times, they themselves fall asleep and would have to wake up just to go their own rooms, at which point their sleep's already disrupted. Their evening sleep's practically ruined by then. It also makes the child dependent on the presence of the parents to fall and stay asleep, which is a behavior that actually needs to be corrected.

That's why some parents choose to let their toddler or baby sleep in their own bed until they're old enough to sleep on their own. It minimizes the disruption in their sleep. And most kids are able to adjust well to sleeping in their own beds and rooms as they reach a certain age so this strategy is one that many parents have adopted.

There's no right or wrong between the two. As the parent of your toddler, you're in the best position to see which option is best for your child, especially when it comes to helping him get deep and restful sleep.

Let Your Child Know What Will Happen

For this, you can do something fun. Pretend to act out a mini-play using props such as your child's stuffed toys and if none are available, use his pillows. Here, one of the "characters" will play the part of putting off bedtime. Using the props, act out what will actually happen as part of the pre-sleep routine.

For example, you act out the part of the "parents" by saying "It's bed time!" Then, you can act out the baby's role (represented by one of the props) asking to be cuddled or rocked to sleep in reaction to the call to go to bed. Next, you also act out the parents' response to the request where they say "No, we will just hold you as you go to bed." Then, you can act out the part where the baby prop cries, to which the parents respond by holding the child until he eventually settles down and sleeps.

When acting out the firmness part of the skit, it's important to do so in a calm and loving manner that firmly insists that the child should already sleep. Over time, your child can identify with the "baby" prop and sees that it eventually goes to sleep. The key here is to show through your skit that the parents always assure the child that they will always be there for him.

Waking Up At Night

As your child learns how to sleep by himself, waking up in the middle of the night tends to become less frequent because he will have grown accustomed to not having you or your spouse around when he wakes up in the middle of the night. While your child's still getting to that point, it's highly possible that he will still wake up at night, especially when he still needs you around in order to fall asleep.

During those times, it may be easier to just let your toddler climb on your bed to sleep with you as he still hasn't learned to fall asleep on his own without having to be held. Otherwise, it may just lead to frequently waking up at night. As he starts becoming accustomed to falling asleep just being with you and not touching you, he'll eventually be able to go back to sleep on his own at night without need to wake you up.

If at that point your child does wake you up and needs you at night, then you can start discouraging such behavior by taking your child back to his bed and sitting beside him while he falls back to sleep.

If you're a mom and you're nursing your toddler, it's alright to nurse him at night for as long as you're okay with it. But, as with many other toddlers, it's possible for your child to wake up all night just to ask for milk. In a case such as this, I advise that you start night-weaning your toddler already, which shouldn't adversely affect your nursing relationship. Just ensure that during your child's waking hours, there are lots of nursing opportunities to make up for the lack of milk in the evenings.

One of the best ways to break off the nursing habit at night if you're a mom, is to ask for help from your husband or partner by sending him to your child at night when he wakes up. And if you're strong enough to enforce this strictly, by informing your toddler during the day that you can't come to the rescue at night because you need to rest and that only your husband or partner can do that, your child will slowly learn to accept that and comply. The key here is someone is there to give your child comfort in the night time waking moments.

When Your Child Cries

It's challenging for your child to learn new sleeping habits. It's possible he may cry and emotionally blackmail you into reverting back to the previous arrangement. Just look at it as your child's way of expressing his fear of being away from or sleeping without you. It's normal for your child to feel like he is being neglected when this happens, and being cognizant of this can help you understand and deal with him much better.

What you need to do at this point is to simply listen to your child's expression of fear and acknowledge his fear by saying something like "I understand you're worried. Don't worry, I'll be very close to you and will always come to your side if you call for help. And I know you're capable of falling asleep even if I'm not beside you." When you allow your child to just cry out his fear to you, you help the child to fall asleep easily because that allows him to experience the fears he's been trying to shoo away. The difference between this and just letting him cry his lungs out is that, in this case, you don't let your child face those fears alone but with the assurance that you're always there to help him face those fears. This makes your child more and more confident and eventually, those fears will go away.

When your child goes hysterical, it's a different story that requires a slightly different approach. Just hold him during such episodes, which is fine as long as you are there with your child. Don't rush your child into being quiet and hurry into moving away as fast as possible. It may be more than your child is capable of handling.

Crying can still allow your child to fall asleep but hysteria's an altogether different matter. If at this point, if your child is still majorly upset with attempts to let him fall asleep on his own, you can always postpone and try again when he's a bit older or you can simply slow down the pace at which you're trying to get him there.

Here's an example of how it can pan out. Supposing your toddler is accustomed to falling asleep while you rock him. You can start by simply putting your child on the bed and tell him that starting from now, you will all fall asleep on the bed.

Or a gentler version could work like this. Continue rocking him to sleep while seated on a chair but this time, only until almost asleep – still a bit awake. At that point, stand up and continue rocking your child in your arms. After a while, stop the rocking and be still. When your child seems to be comfortable with being still and is still somewhat awake, but almost asleep, lower him into the bed or crib. If your child protests, pick him up again and rock for a short while and then stop. Put him back on the bed again and repeat if your child protests. With enough repetition, your child will learn to fall asleep without protest when you put him down on the bed or crib. If you find this a wee bit too laborious or cumbersome, just keep in mind that it will eventually be worth it when your child finally learns to sleep on his own as a result of your patience and perseverance.

Could this crying be traumatic for your child over the long run? Not if you do it right and don't rush it. Remember, crying is your child's way of expressing his fears and if you allow him to cry while being close by to make him feel secure in your love and support through touching and verbal reassuring, trauma is highly unlikely. Just don't force your child to "get it" quickly or at your preferred pace.

Just keep in mind that the first several nights are the most challenging ones. Your child will most probably protest with much vitality and passion when you start saying "no" to his crying requests, especially if he's already been accustomed to you rocking him to sleep. It's normal because at his age, your child has no idea of what life is like without you rocking him to sleep, which makes crying out of fear a very normal and expected reaction.

But as you continue to consistently act out the new routine by staying beside him, by acting a mini-skit with stuffed toys or pillows, and holding and reassuring your child, lying down and sleeping independently will eventually happen. At first, it may take over an hour for your child to fall asleep but you can expect - within a week or two - that your child will be able to fall asleep within minutes after being put back down.

Recognize Your Toddler's Bravery

When your child makes progress in terms of sleeping alone, whether big or small, don't let the opportunity to commend and recognize him for those accomplishments pass by. Motivation will go a long way towards encouraging your child to continue and eventually learn to sleep by himself, which can be a very significant accomplishment for him. When you act out your mini-skit with the stuffed toys or pillows, make sure that the skit includes the "parents" commending and recognizing the "baby's" progress. You can further motivate your child with appropriate rewards that he will appreciate, such as a toy, extended playtime, or his favorite treat.

A gradually progressing system of helping your child sleep soundly on his own is one that gives your child a deep sense of security and the opportunity to learn how to fall asleep by himself. Just continue to patiently and lovingly work with your toddler towards helping him achieve sleeping independence.

Chapter 4: 12 to 18 Month-Old Toddlers

In the previous chapter, we discussed general techniques to help your child go to sleep. In this and the next three chapters, we'll take a look at more specific ways of helping your child go to sleep: according to age and number (multiple toddlers, e.g., twins, triplets, or 2 or more toddlers of roughly the same age). Let's begin with the toddlers 12 to 18 months old.

For toddlers within this age range, the most common sleeping issue is waking frequently in the middle of the night. Some toddlers of this age bracket can wake up as frequent as five times in an evening. But the real concern here isn't why he wakes up frequently during the night but whether or not he can go back to sleep. And if not, why?

If, during this age bracket, your toddler's still unable to go back sleep by himself, it's highly likely that he's unable to do the complete bed routine by himself at this point. At this point, one of the challenges you may face with your toddler is that he's already able to tell that you will leave the room as soon as he falls asleep. Because he still doesn't know how his sleeping life will be without you or your spouse beside him or close by, he probably won't want to sleep just yet. And he will probably make that desire known by crying.

So what are you to do? One thing you can do is to train your child to make new sleep-related associations other than you leaving immediately the moment he dozes off. If you're able to do this, you don't need to get out of bed several times during the night. To make this work, you'll first have to ensure you've already established and are running a consistent bedtime ritual for your child.

You can also try seeing the evening from the eyes of your child. Go to his room and try to think about how your child sees the room at two in the morning. The key is to make the bedroom look the same all throughout the night. Unless you're open to sitting beside him to sing, you should be out of the room before your child dozes off so that when he wakes up in the middle of the night, it won't look and feel much different from before he dozed off.

And you may need some props to make this happen. One way to do it is by turning on an electric fan that can drown out most of the ambient sounds that can be heard in your child's room.

You will also need to work on developing your poker face. If and when your child calls out to you in the middle of the night, simply check the room and assure your child everything's okay. Refrain from playing, cuddling or hanging out for too long, which will require you to be both gentle and firm. The point of this exercise is for your child to associate inconvenience or an unrewarding experience with calling out for you in the middle of the night just to go back to bed.

You can also start teaching your child delayed gratification during these moments. As the night wears on, slowly extend the time that passes between him calling you and you going to his room. Let 5 minutes pass at the start, then 10 minutes, then 15 and so on. Allow your child several days to adjust fully every time you extend your response time. Give your child several weeks to establish this new association and develop the habit of being able to go back to sleep on his own as well.

Chapter 5: 18 Month to 3 Year-Old Toddlers

During this age bracket, you may be subjected to a new round of challenges when it comes to settling your toddler down in the evening as well as making him sleep through the night. Some of the more common issues that you may face during this age range include evening anxieties, bedtime struggles and transferring beds. Let's talk about how to handle these in more detail.

Evening Anxieties

Your toddler may start feeling anxious about several things at night, including being left alone in the room in the dark, fearful of monsters beneath his bed and being scared of the dark itself. When your toddler expresses his fear of these things, just reassure him that it's perfectly safe in the bedroom where everything's well. But more importantly, reassure him that you are always nearby so when he calls for help, you will be there.

There are other ways you can help make him feel less anxious about the dark. You can leave his bedroom door ajar with the lights outside still on, or leave a dim nightlight on in the room. These are small things that may give him the courage to face the evening anxieties and sleep well and easy.

At this point, your toddler's very active and developing imagination may also result in occasional bad dreams or nightmares. When your toddler wakes up screaming or crying as a result of these, immediately come to his side and be sure to comfort your toddler until calmed down. If the dream is vivid and he can remember it, ask if your child wants to talk about it.

If not, just continue reassuring him that it was just a dream and that all's well and fine until he gets settled in once again.

Quite often, nightmares happen during the latter part of his evening sleeping time. It's because at this time, your toddler's chances of experiencing REM or rapid eye movement dream sleep is at its highest. If the nightmares continue occurring frequently, it would be wise for you to figure out other possible sources of anxiety. It may just be separation anxiety, overtiredness, or a scary story he may have remembered that are causing nightmares.

Apart from nightmares, it's possible for your child to experience night terrors during this age bracket too, which manifest themselves in the form of screaming or crying during sleep coupled with a great sense of confusion and disorientation. These are different from nightmares in that these usually happen during the earliest part of deep sleep, often referred to as non-REM sleep. When these happen, your toddler may scream, cry out, and even thrash out while half-asleep and half-awake. He may not even recognize you when you try to give comfort and reassurance. When this happens, don't attempt to wake your toddler up – do so only when it's clear that he may get hurt in the process. Just stand or sit with your toddler until it passes, after which you can gently usher him back to sleep.

While it can be quite alarming or frightening for a parent to witness a toddler going through a night terror, rest assured that, save for extreme cases, it's not harmful to your child. Chances are, he won't even remember a single detail about it in the morning.

Your child may be more prone to experiencing these when he's anxious or overtired. To address any potential sources of anxiety, consider having a conversation with your child to find out if indeed, something's bothering him. Quite frequently, simply being able to share fears or worries is enough to ease anxieties and minimize or even stop night terrors from happening. To address the concern of overtiredness, it's paramount that you're able to get him to bed on time every night for consistently deep and refreshing sleep. Otherwise, the lack of sleep may exacerbate his already being overtired due to lack of quality sleep.

Bedtime Struggles

Another common sleeping-related challenge for parents of toddlers in this age bracket is the tendency for children to struggle against being ushered into sleeping at night. These struggles may include stalling tactics such as asking for one more bedtime story, another glass of milk or water and another lullaby.

So how can you best handle these struggling tactics and usher your child consistently into Wonderland? One way is to plan ahead by anticipating potential "requests" your toddler may make. For example, you can take him to the toilet, change his diaper, or ensure that he already has a drink of milk or water – all before settling down to sleep. You can also make your toddler choose 2 to 3 bedtime stories prior to settling down and there's no harm in reading him another story or enjoying extended cuddling time for as long you're clear and firm about sleeping in on time.

Keep in mind that if you let your toddler sleep too much during the day, he will have a hard time sleeping at night, which may explain why you are struggling in your attempts to make him sleep at a certain time in the evening. To minimize the impact of over-napping, make sure that any naps shouldn't extend past 3 in the afternoon. Doing this will significantly increase the chances of your toddler being "tired enough" to sleep on time at night.

Transferring Beds

From ages 2 to 3 years old, toddlers are highly likely to be ready to make the big transition to a big bed. Your toddler may have already grown to be too big for his existing cot. He may already be potty training at this point and moving to a big bed can provide easy access to the potty in the evening.

If you're also expecting a new baby at this time, your toddler's cot may be needed shortly for the expected infant. If so, it's better if you can move your toddler to the big bed at least 8 weeks before your due date. Doing so will help give your toddler enough time to get settled in the new bed, which will keep him from resenting the new sibling because of the impression that the newborn is taking over his cot at his expense.

For an easier transition period for your toddler, position the big bed where the cot used to be if space permits it. That should give your toddler some semblance of familiarity even in the new bed. You can also let your toddler sleep on the new bed using the old cot blanket for a few days or weeks, again just to give him a sense of familiarity and security in the new sleeping environment.

Make sure that the big bed is equipped with guardrails, which will keep your toddler from accidentally falling off the bed. You can try to install a stair gate outside your toddler's bedroom or at the top of your home's stairs – if it has stairs – if you're worried about your toddler exploring outside the bedroom in the night. Lastly, make sure the room is toddler-proofed. At your toddler's age, his curiosity is growing in leaps and bounds, which can significantly increase the likelihood of accidental injuries.

To reinforce the new sleeping behavior, be sure to lavish lots of praise on your toddler every time he is able to stay in the new bed all through his bedtime. When he gets up from the bed, which is normal within the first few days, given that it's an adjustment period, just put your toddler back to bed and settle him down again. Calmly, but firmly, tell him it's time for sleep and you must leave the room immediately. Just give it time and your toddler will eventually get used to this new sleeping routine.

Chapter 6: 3 to 6 Year-Old Toddlers

This age bracket is when your preschool toddler starts to crave attention, which may lead to him frequently getting out of bed or calling you back into the room so he can get "enough" of you. Fortunately, you can use this craving for attention to their advantage as well as yours and make them sleep.

Stage It

One way to do this is to set up your appearance in stages. Right after saying goodnight to your toddler, tell him that you'll be back for another short story or goodnight kiss in 5 minutes – if he will stay in bed and keep quiet. Just repeat this practice over and over, gradually increasing the time before your return from the initial 5 minutes. Over the course of 1 week, increase the return intervals and reduce the number of times you return. The secret lies in going back to give your toddler that attention he craves. But if you do this, you must be careful to keep your word.

For some clingy toddlers, a little creativity may be in order. You can feign forgetting to do a household chore such as turning off the TV, turning on the dishwasher, or loading the washing machine. As you go out to do the chore, you can reassure your child that you'll be back right after you're done with the "chore" or leave a dim nightlight on for reassurance. You can also leave an item you were holding in the room, such as a magazine or an apron. Doing this can help your toddler see there's something you'll have to come back for in the room after your chore, which will make him confident that you will really come back. If your toddler's still awake by the time you get back into the room, praise him for quietly staying on the bed, and give another goodnight kiss.

Leveling

You can also try to be gentle yet honest with your child about the potential benefits and consequences of sleeping in on time and staying in bed the whole evening, and of not being able to do so, respectively. For example, you can tell your child how much nicer mommy or daddy will be in the morning if you can get uninterrupted sleep as a result of your toddler staying in bed the whole night and not interrupting you. Just make sure you make good on such promises by, in this example, smothering your toddler with kisses and hugs as soon as he sees you in the morning. Doing so reinforces the behavior by teaching him that there's an effective way to get the attention he craves, and that's by sleeping in on time and staying in bed the whole evening.

Night Terrors

Similar to the previous age bracket, night terrors are frequent in toddlers of this age group. These normally peak at this age bracket and are believed to affect 1 in every 20 kids. These usually happen within the first 2 hours of deep sleep and would usually begin with your toddler screaming. It's even possible that during these episodes, your toddler may sweat, breathe fast, and flail – or even jump out of bed!

As mentioned earlier, night terrors seem scarier than they actually are – they're harmless most of the time. The only thing you should do is to ensure your child's safety when these things happen and do nothing more – not even waking him up.

Chapter 7:   Putting Twins or Siblings to Sleep

It's one thing to put a toddler to sleep and keep him asleep during the evening. It's different if you're talking about 2 or more; twins, triplets, quadruplets or close-aged siblings. Let's talk about how to handle this unique sleeping situation well.

Sleeping Schedule

Let's face it, one of the advantages of your children entering the toddler stage is that they may enjoy a high likelihood of sleeping throughout the evening, which allows you to experience the same. Why? It's because most kids sleep between 10 to 12 hours nightly after turning 1, and enjoy periodic naps during the day.

On the 2nd year, your toddlers' nightly sleeping schedule isn't likely to change significantly. The daytime nap periods may be where significant changes may happen. While infants normally sleep on an intermittent basis during the day, a 1 ½ year old toddler would only require a 2-hour nap after lunch.

With this, it can be quite challenging for you to implement a sleeping schedule that can meet the changing needs for 2 or more toddlers simultaneously. This is a period that will require much flexibility and patience from you. As such, one of the best ways to manage this is to keep your toddlers on the same sleeping routine and schedule as much as possible. However, you must be aware of each toddler's individual sleeping needs as you do this. The hierarchy of priorities would still be needs over schedule, so fit them on the same schedules only to the extent that it doesn't compromise each of your toddlers' needs.

Bed versus Crib

Twins or triplets, on average, tend to stay in cribs longer than single infants. However, you should still be open to the possibility of moving them into big beds at the same stage of infancy as single infants are. Just bear in mind that doing so can be very challenging, particularly when you remove the restrictions that kept them inside the crib previously. When such restrictions are removed, it's highly likely for your toddlers to mess around with the room's contents during the night.

You may be tempted to think of just putting off transferring them to a big bed for as long as possible to minimize the chances of this happening. But keep in mind that the crib isn't always going to be the safest sleep haven for your multi-toddlers. There will come a time when the crib may actually be more dangerous. It's because when they reach the age of ability and extreme curiosity, it's highly likely for them to attempt to climb out of the crib, which puts them at high risk of a serious fall and the injuries that may result from it.

If you choose to put off the transfer for as long as possible, one risk reducing measure is to remove any object from the crib that your toddlers can use as a platform on which to step as a means of climbing out of the crib. These may include toys, pillows or bumper pads. You can also set the crib's mattress as low into the crib as possible to maximize the height of the railings and minimize the risk of your toddlers being able to climb from them.

The inevitable, however, will come. Your toddlers will eventually need to say goodbye to the comfort of their cribs. Because of this, you must plan ahead to ensure a smooth and safe transition. Fortunately, toddler beds are gaining in popularity throughout the years, which have made them a very good option for regular cribs and regular beds. While toddler beds are proportionally sized to accommodate young children, they can be a bit costly to buy, considering that if you have twins, you'll need 2 of them, more so if you have triplets or even quadruplets!

If you find it too expensive to get toddler beds, there's a good DIY alternative: use regular beds without the frame or rails. You can just position the box springs and mattresses on the ground to provide low-height and safer toddler beds that you can eventually reassemble back into regular ones when your toddlers are old enough for regular beds.

Safe Sleep

Your toddlers will have much access to the stuff in their environment when out of their cribs. An even bigger concern is that it comes with an increasing sense of curiosity that can make them touch things that shouldn't be touched or eat stuff that mustn't be ingested. You must make sure to childproof your home, if not the toddlers' bedroom, which is of highest priority! Anything that looks like and can be a toddler hazard is a hazard – remove them immediately!

Together or Apart?

As you consider transitioning your toddlers to beds, another thing you'll need to consider is whether or not they should continue being in the same room. While being together and apart both have their share of advantages and disadvantages, what's important is to know your toddlers' needs and which options are best for meeting those needs. It's possible that being separated, multiple toddlers may feel the need to more frequently get up at night as an attempt to be reunited with their separated sibling or siblings. It's also possible that your toddlers are introverts or loners, who may be more comfortable sleeping without the unnecessary distractions and disruptions from the other siblings. So figure out your toddlers' preferences and, if budget allows, choose accordingly.

Routines

Consistency helps embed routines and sleeping habits deep into your multiple toddlers' psyches and help them to be expectant about sleeping time. Just repeat the same routines and patterns night in and night out, from taking a bath, brushing their teeth, changing into their jammies, you telling them stories, giving them goodnight hugs and kisses, and turning off the lights. And more than just the same routine, ensure that you do them at the same time at night as much as possible. Consistency in sleeping routines can help promote good sleep behavior.

Manage the Environment

The bedroom environment is a crucial factor in setting the right mood for your toddlers when it comes to sleeping at night. For this, you must create an environment that's relaxing and calm – a soft environment if you will. This includes making the lights dim, talking in a much softer tone of voice, and removing anything that can be stressful or distracting to your toddlers.

Independence

Remember that the ultimate goal is to enable your multiple toddlers to put themselves to sleep. You shouldn't condition them to need your presence in the room just to doze off. As soon as you see them settled in and comfortable, leave the room immediately. Thus, it won't be a wise idea to lie down with your multiple toddlers every night, which can only fortify their clinginess or sense of dependence on you. Over time, you should cultivate in them a sense of sleeping independence.

Chapter 8: The (Sleep) Walking Toddler

Compared to adults, sleepwalking is actually more common in children, especially toddlers. By the time children turn into teenagers, most of them outgrow sleepwalking. It can also be hereditary so if you or your spouse or partner is known to have sleepwalked in the past, it's not far-fetched to think your toddler may sleepwalk too.

More than just genetics, sleepwalking in toddlers may also be due to fatigue, sleep deprivation, inconsistent sleeping habits, sickness, medicines or stress.

Manifestations

More than just walking around while asleep, which is clearly the most obvious sign that your toddler is sleepwalking, other symptoms or manifestations include talking in their sleep, difficulty waking up, being dazed, clumsiness, unresponsiveness during conversations, and going through repeated actions while sitting up in bed. A popular misconception about sleepwalkers is that a child's eyes are always closed, which isn't always the case. It's possible to sleepwalk with eyes wide open, where toddlers see things differently, e.g., they think they're in another part of the house or in another place.   Sleepwalking may also be accompanied by night terrors, enuresis (also known as bed wetting), and sleep apnea (short breathing pauses during sleep).

Is It Dangerous For Your Toddler?

In and by itself, it isn't. Sleepwalking isn't a disorder or a sign of such. In fact, it isn't even a symptom of psychological or emotional issues. What can make it dangerous, however, is the fact that when your toddlers sleepwalk, they're not aware of what they're doing, which puts them at risk of doing something potentially harmful like walking out of an open window or falling down a flight of stairs.

Keeping Your Sleepwalking Toddler Safe

As mentioned earlier, it's the fact that your toddlers aren't aware of what they're doing during sleepwalking episodes that make potentially dangerous. Thus, you need to implement measures to ensure their safety should they unconsciously decide to go for a night stroll in their rooms or throughout the house.

- Do not attempt to wake your toddler up as he sleepwalks. This will only scare your child and make it even harder for him to go back to sleep. What you should do instead is to calmly and gently lead your toddler back to bed.
- Make sure all the windows are locked in your toddler's bedroom and all over the house. Consider installing additional locks or even child-proof locks on your home's doors and windows. Make sure keys are well out of reach of your toddlers.
- Never let your toddler sleep on a bunk bed, which can put him at risk of falling badly to the floor.
- Make sure there aren't any sharp or fragile objects around your toddler's bed and be sure to keep dangerous items far from his reach.
- As much as possible, take away any obstacles inside the toddler's room to minimize his risk of tripping or stumbling. In particular, make sure the floor's clutter free.
- Put safety gates at the top of your stairs and outside your toddler's bedroom.

Helping Your Sleepwalking Toddler

If your toddler's sleepwalking adventures don't happen often, don't make him lethargic or sluggish during the day, or put him in harm's way, you don't have to do anything about them. Otherwise, it's best for you to see a doctor, especially if there's a possibility of it being accompanied by breathing difficulties or reflux.

If it's just about frequent sleepwalking, many child experts suggest conducting what's referred to as scheduled awakening. This option is one where you disrupt your toddler's sleep cycle frequently enough to put a stop to the frequent sleepwalking adventures. If symptoms persist, a doctor could prescribe medication for sleep.

You can also help minimize or even stop sleepwalking incidents by helping your toddler relax in the evening prior to going to bed by listening to soothing sounds or using a white noise machine to play soothing and relaxing white noise in the background.

Do not encourage your kids to drink so much water or milk prior to sleeping to minimize the chances of sleepwalking. Also, ensure that they pee before going to bed every night. Why? A loaded bladder increases the likelihood of your toddler sleepwalking.

Chapter 9: Travelling Toddlers and Sleep

Going out of town for family vacations is one of the best ways to create beautiful memories for you and your kids. However, it can also be a particularly challenging time when it comes to making your toddler sleep. In this chapter, we'll take a look at different ways you can help your toddler get good sleep even while on vacation away from home.

It Starts At the Beginning

When going out of town for a family vacation, it's best to go well rested. Any form of long distance travel – be it by train, plane, or car – can deprive anybody of a decent shuteye but it can be especially stressful for toddlers rather than older people. This is because toddlers – compared to older people – tend to pile up sleep debts or deficits much faster.

Before going on a long trip, make sure that your toddler gets enough rest and sleep beforehand. On the days and nights preceding your trip, let your toddler have the opportunity to take restorative naps during the day and ample sleep at night. Toddlers and infants with fully loaded sleep tanks are able to adapt much better to temporary changes in schedule brought about by out of town vacations, as well as to the resulting sleep loss.

Work The Itinerary around the Toddler's Sleeping Time

Kids are naturally stimulated and excited by the mere planning of a vacation or travel. Thus, it's hard for them to sleep on the way to your family's vacation destination. To work around this, try planning your trip's departure and arrival schedules around your toddler's nap times, whenever possible.

If your toddler still naps before lunch, plan to leave for your vacation destination after your toddler's morning nap. Keep in mind that of all the daytime naps your toddler can take, it's the first one in the morning that tends to be most helpful in curbing overtiredness throughout the day. It's also the most restorative of the daytime naps.

When possible, time your destination arrival before your toddler's normal bedtime. Taking naps on the road or in flight is never as restful as real naps on a bed and as such, your toddler would need to recoup the lost quality sleep in transit in the evening. Arriving at the destination before his usual sleeping time minimizes sleeping disruptions and allows him to recoup lost naps during travel by sleeping at an earlier time at night.

Sleeping Environment

Another very important factor to manage and plan for when it comes to travelling and ensuring your toddler's sleep is the sleeping environment. Even for a full-grown adult, having to drastically change the sleeping environment can wreak havoc on one's sleeping pattern, which is the case when travelling out of town. Can you imagine how much this affects your toddler?

If you have the budget for it, go for a large room that can provide you with extra space for a pull out mattress or a crib. That can give you the privilege of enjoying the night as your toddler sleeps nearby. If you can get a room with a kitchen, you can save more money by having a place to store snacks and milk that you take along.

But if you don't have a budget for a big room and you're stuck in a one-room unit, don't worry. You can be as creative as you want and figure out how to fit a small bed or crib into the room that is separate from you and your spouse or partner's bed. A good space for it could be a large closet (kept open of course), a hallway, or even the bathroom. It may also help to rearrange the room's furniture or hang a sheet from the room's ceiling to create a semblance of physical separation from your toddler and continue the sleeping habits and routine that you follow at home as much as possible.

What if your toddler eventually finds his way to your hotel bed, which isn't an ideal scenario? Don't worry about it and how it can affect how he will transition back into his separate bed when you are at home after the vacation. Tell him during the trip that this "accommodation" is just for this trip and that when the family returns home, he will be sleeping back in his own bed. By frequently reminding your toddler about this during the trip and during the ride back home, you minimize the risk of your toddler backsliding to join you back in bed at home.

If needed and if possible, reserve (buy or rent) the beds you may need for your toddler on your vacation. If you frequently visit your in-laws or family in another state or country, ask them to rent or borrow a crib that's portable. If you plan to stay in a hotel or motel, call them ahead of time to ensure that the extra pullout mattress or crib will be available when you get there. And if you're bringing your own family car, you can bring your own foldable bed, sleeping bag, or crib.

Rehearse

Because out of town trips tend to be disruptive to any person's routine, regardless if you'll be staying at a relative's or a friend's house or in a hotel, it's important to rehearse what your toddler's sleeping routine will be out of town several days before leaving the house. The key is to keep the routine disruptions to your toddler's sleeping routines to a minimum. By rehearsing the vacation sleeping routine ahead of time, your toddler can have some semblance of familiarity even on the road. It can help him sleep easily.

How does a rehearsal work? If you plan to bring a portable crib or a travel bed, let your toddler sleep in it for consecutive nights prior to leaving for your family trip. You can also have a nice little chat with your toddler about your family's travel plans, which include possible sleeping arrangements.

Things to Bring

Another way to increase your child's chances of sleeping soundly while on vacation is to bring the right stuff along for the trip, i.e., useful sleeping accessories such as:

- White Noise Generating App: An app like Relax Melodies can be a very useful relaxation agent for your toddler, as it can be so relaxing and soothing for him. White noise can help lessen or even dampen the presence of undesirable ambient noise, which can disrupt your toddler's sleep.
- Your Toddler's Favorite Stuffed Toy or Pillows: Just keep it to one or two, though it's tempting to bring the whole crew along for the ride.
- Your Own Bed Or Crib Sheets: Using familiar sheets on the bed where your toddler will eventually sleep can help provide some level of familiarity to make him feel relaxed and comfortable enough to have a good night's sleep.
- Painter's Tape and Black Plastic Bags: These can help you manage your toddler's sleeping environment by serving as good substitute for blackout curtains while on the road. Remember, darkness is important for a good night's rest as it helps promote release of the sleep hormone

melatonin.

- Strollers: As travelling becomes more and more unpredictably delayed these days, having a stroller along can help your toddler get much needed shut eye wherever you and the family may get stuck such as the airport, bus station, or the dock. It'll also give you a much easier time carrying your toddler around as it has wheels, instead of having to physically carry them around on your shoulders while they nap.

Do the Routines

Just because you and your toddler aren't at home doesn't mean you can't continue with your usual bedtime routines. This is where consistency becomes even more important as a means of strengthening already established habits and minimize risks for backsliding into old ones. Stick to your normal routine on vacation, it shouldn't be too different to being at home. The key is predictability and consistency. And if your toddler's already accustomed to the routines, then continuing them away from home can signal his body to sleep at the same time as at home.

Nap As Frequently As Needed

Regardless of whether you're on vacation at your in-laws or walking around in Lego Land, the temptation to ditch your toddler's usual daytime naps can be very strong. But if you give in to the temptation, you may eventually regret it when your toddler becomes agitated or cranky due to the major disruption in his sleeping routine or schedule.

If a particularly busy day on vacation required your toddler to skip a nap or two, make sure that the next days won't deprive him of such naps again. During the remaining days, schedule your activities in a way that you won't deny your toddler those crucial daytime naps that have become part of his good sleeping routine. But if it's unavoidable, try to compensate by going to bed earlier in the evening.

Remember, the more you allow your toddler's sleep deficit to accumulate, the more you increase his risk of him melting down and making life difficult for all the members of the family. So be as flexible as possible and work around your toddler's daytime nap requirements. Even a simple nap inside the car or a stroller can be enough for your toddler to get much needed naps.

Time Zones

If your vacation involves traveling to places in a different time zone, you must move your schedule to match that time zone as early as possible. And when coming back home, do the same for a few days prior to doing so. Move your schedule back to your home's time zone.

If you're travelling for just a couple of days, it may be okay to just stay on your time zone. But if you plan to travel for a week or more outside of your time zone, then it's best to start shifting your toddler's sleeping time zones one week out from departure. Start by shifting in 15-minute increments until you're able to completely adapt to your vacation destination place's time zone. Expect to successfully do this within 4 to 7 days.

Should you decide it's a bit too cumbersome to start the gradual shift days prior to departure, try to shift your child's sleeping routines according to the new time zone as soon as you get there. You can either wake him up as close as possible to the sleeping time equivalent of the new time zone or simply let him be if he wakes up earlier than usual in the new time zone and chooses to perform the sleeping routines at the usual time as back home. And to help your toddler transition well in terms of sleeping schedule, use bright lights in the morning and dim lights in the evening to shift his sleep or circadian rhythm cycle.

Be Firm but Not Strict

Remember the point of going on a vacation, which is for the family to enjoy bonding together. As such, don't be too strict about sleeping routines while on vacation. True, it'd be good to stick as close as possible to said routines but you also have to remember that being on vacation outside your home, you don't have access to the same comforts, structure, and facilities as you do back home. And that makes it very challenging to perfectly stick to the "rules."

Just be firm in the sense that you don't let your toddler stray too far away from his usual sleeping routine. For as long as he's generally within the routine, give him a break, if only during the vacation. When you get back home, then that's the time to be strict about routines.

Resume As Soon As Possible

As soon as you get back home from vacation, do your best to resume the sleeping routines completely as soon as possible. That can be the most challenging part of coming back home but persevere, and be firm about it with your toddler. If you don't, you'll practically have to start all over again.

Conclusion

Thank you for buying this book. I hope that it's able to help you learn how to deal much better with your toddlers, particularly when it comes to going to sleep. And while I'm glad that you want to learn how to do that successfully every night, knowing is only half the battle. The other half is action – the application of knowledge.

To this end, I want to strongly encourage you to start applying the things you learned in this book as soon as possible. It doesn't have to be all at the same time – just take, pardon the pun, toddler steps. If you continue putting off any action, you increase the risk of not applying anything you learned and therefore, risk not being able to help your toddler to consistently go to sleep easily and enjoy refreshing night rests. So start with even just one lesson you learned in this book as soon as possible.

Here's to your toddler's – and yours as well – deep and restful sleep! Cheers!

Finally, if you enjoyed this book, then I'd like to ask you for a favor, would you be kind enough to leave a review for this book on Amazon? It'd be greatly appreciated!

Thank you and good luck!